The Dash Diet

Everything You Need to Know and 50
Incredible Dash Diet Recipes

AUTHOR: REBECCA BELLIS

Legal & Disclaimer

The information contained in this book and its contents is not designed to replace or take the place of any form of medical or professional advice; and is not meant to replace the need for independent medical, financial, legal or other professional advice or services, as may be required. The content and information in this book have been provided for educational and entertainment purposes only.

The content and information contained in this book have been compiled from sources deemed reliable, and it is accurate to the best of the Author's knowledge, information, and belief. However, the Author cannot guarantee its accuracy and validity and cannot be held liable for any errors and omissions. Further, changes are periodically made to this book as and when needed. Where appropriate and necessary, you must consult a professional (including but not limited to your doctor, attorney, financial advisor or such other professional advisor) before using any of the suggested remedies, techniques, or information in this book.

Upon using the contents and information contained in this book, you agree to hold harmless the Author from and against any damages, costs, and expenses, including any legal fees potentially resulting from the application of any of the information provided by this book. This disclaimer applies to any loss, damages or injury caused by the use and application, whether directly or indirectly, of any advice or information

Contents

Chapter 6. Dash Diet Snack and Appetizer Recipes 102

Conclusion 122

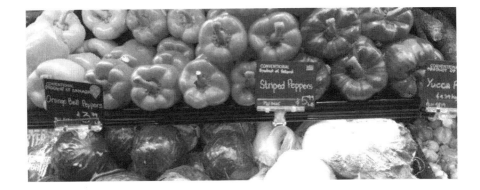

Preface

Are you constantly searching for healthy ways to improve your health and look amazing?

Are you sick and tired of all those miraculous diets that promise you results in no time but turn out to be fake?

Well, today your search is over! I searched and discovered the best diet you can use to become a healthy person!

It's the Dash diet!

This is much more than a simple diet! It's a healthy lifestyle that will make you a new person! It's the best diet to lower your blood pressure and improve your appearance!

Are you curious to learn more?

Then you are in the right place! All you have to do is to get your hands on *The Dash Diet: Everything You Need to Know and 50 Incredible Dash Diet Recipes*!

This unbelievable book provides you with all the information you need about the Dash diet and 50 incredible recipes you can make!

The Dash Diet: Everything You Need to Know and 50 Incredible Dash Diet Recipes is extremely well organized, all the information is accessible, and all the recipes are easy to make at home! This book will make you fall in love with the Dash diet and it will soon become part of your life!

Get a copy of *The Dash Diet: Everything You Need to Know and 50 Incredible Dash Diet Recipes* today and enjoy a new life!

Chapter 1. Everything You Need to Know About the Dash Diet

What is the Dash Diet?

The Dash Diet stands for Dietary Approaches to Stop Hypertension. This is much more than a simple diet. It's actually a well-respected lifestyle these days. It's not some miraculous weight loss diet! It's a healthy way of life!

The Dash Diet was designed to lower blood pressure and reduce the risk of heart diseases. Also, this healthy diet is much healthier than standard diets and it's been known to bring many other health benefits as well.

Among the health benefits of this diet are:

- Decreased risk of cancer
- Decreased risk of diabetes
- Lower cholesterol levels
- Decreased risk of stroke
- Healthy weight loss
- Decreased risk of osteoporosis

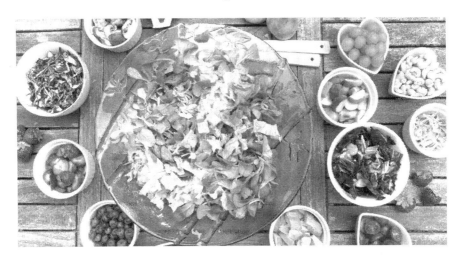

This diet's main focus is to help you reduce the sodium intake and start eating healthier foods that contain important elements and vitamins. The Dash diet will reduce your blood pressure by 10-20 points and you will see amazing transformation in no time.

Does that sound amazing or what?

There are two Dash Diet options. The best thing to do is consult your doctor before starting either one.

During the first Dash Diet option, you can consume up to 2300 mg of sodium per day.

The second option is a lower sodium version during which you can only consume up to 1500 mg of sodium/day.

Experts in the field discovered the second Dash Diet version is better for lowering blood pressure, but both of them are great!

For you to understand better what this translates into, take a look at the general Dash Diet daily nutrient goals. This will help you develop your meal plans easier.

Daily Nutrient Goals

Fat: 27% of calories

Carbs: 55%

Protein: 18%

Cholesterol: 150 mg

Sodium: 2300 mg/ 1500 mg

Fiber: 30 g

Remember—this is a general guide to help you adapt easier to your new Dash lifestyle.

What can You Eat on a Dash Diet? What Should You Focus on?

Both versions of the Dash Diet focus on including a lot of veggies, low-fat and non-fat dairy, fruits, whole grains, and lean protein such as poultry, fish, or seafood in your diet. The main thing you need to know is that you not only have to reduce the sodium intake but also the sugar and fat.

You must search for products and ingredients that contain important nutrients such as magnesium, potassium, or calcium.

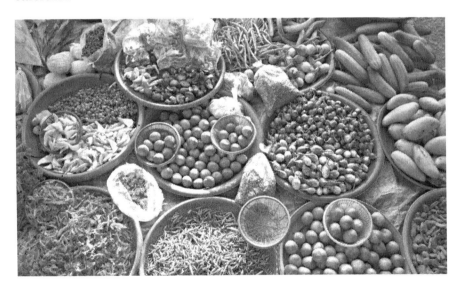

The Daily Recommended Servings for the Standard Dash Diet

This information is based on intense research developed in this particular field.

Grains: 6-8 servings/day

If you are on a Dash Diet, you can consume whole grains such as oats, cereals, quinoa, rice, pasta, or breads! The main thing you must remember is that you mustn't combine them with other products that contain a lot of fat or cholesterol.

Veggies: up to 6 servings/day

If you are on a Dash Diet, you must consume a lot of fresh veggies! You can eat carrots, green beans, celery, turnips, pumpkin, potatoes, spinach, tomatoes, lettuce, kale, and other green vegetables, peppers, etc.

Consume both fresh and frozen veggies, but if you opt for the frozen ones, you should choose those without added salt.

Fruits: up to 6 servings/day

One of the advantages of the Dash Diet is that you can consume a lot of fruits. This includes cherries, dates, bananas, grapefruit, lemons, melons, peaches, pineapple, berries, watermelon, apples, and many others.

Fruits are extremely healthy and contain so many important elements. Your health and appearance will definitely benefit from them.

Dairy: up to 3 servings/day

You can consume low-fat or non-fat dairy milk, cheese, yogurt, buttermilk, and even some butter. The main focus is to include dairy in your daily diet because of the protein and vitamin levels – but make sure you only get the right ones!

Protein: up to 6 servings/day

You can consume meat, poultry, fish, seafood, and even eggs. When it comes to meat, always make sure you only choose lean products, trim the fat, and remove the skin. Meat is a source of important vitamins and healthy fats (fish and seafood) but don't consume more than 6 ounces/day. I recommend you grill, broil, or bake the meat instead of frying it. Frying is an unhealthy cooking method and I suggest you to avoid it.

Nuts, legumes, and seeds: up to 5 servings/ week

You can eat beans, nuts, lentils, chickpeas, almonds, peas, and any other legumes, nuts, and seeds you love. All these contain vitamins and minerals and can improve your overall health and lower your blood pressure.

Fats and Oils: up to 3 servings/day

You can consume olive oil, coconut oil, ghee, and even low-fat butter, but make sure you don't exaggerate. Avoid processed fats and margarine, and only consume limited quantities of shortening or lard.

Sweets: less than 5 servings/week

You can consume some jelly, candy, maple syrup, and even some sugar but take into consideration that the consumption must be limited. You can also consume some fat-free or low-fat graham crackers, low-fat cookies, or sorbets but only every once in a while.

You are allowed to consume some sweets that contain artificial sweeteners as well, like aspartame or sucralose but never exaggerate.

Coffee and Alcohol

It would be best if you limit the consumption of alcohol and coffee during a Dash Diet. Alcohol will increase your blood pressure and prevent you from achieving your goals in terms of weight loss and health. Coffee is not forbidden when you are on a Dash Diet, but consume it in moderation—no more than two servings per day.

Spices and Seasoning

This discussion begins with salt. We are all used to seasoning our meals with salt but if you opt for a Dash Diet, you must change this.

That's what this category is all about! Here are some of the spices I recommend you use instead of salt.

Bay leaves - these are sweet and will enhance the flavor of your meals.

Basil - this is pungent and sweet and it's one of the most popular spices used.

Cinnamon - this is known to lower blood sugar levels and bring flavor to your dishes.

Cardamom - this spice has a peppery flavor and it's mostly used in Indian cuisine.

Ginger powder - you can also use this fresh in many dishes; the best thing is that it adds flavor and taste.

Garlic powder - this replaces salt and it's much healthier.

Pepper - this is a common spice that everyone uses. It's intense and brings more flavor to all your foods.

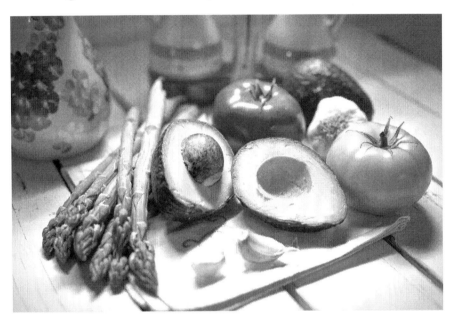

What You Didn't Know About the Dash Diet

This will really surprise you! There are many products that contain hidden sodium levels.

Among these products, you'll find bread and other baked products. You might not know it, but one simple bread slice contains up to 700 mg of sodium. That's a lot, don't you think?

Also muffins, cakes, and even doughnuts contain a lot of sodium.

You may also want to know that some breakfast cereals contain some sodium. So make sure you always check the label before purchasing these products.

Some dairy products can contain salt as well. You might not know this, but cheese contains a lot of salt because it's an important factor in the cheese-making process. Milk contains sodium as well. It might contain up to 120 mg of sodium per ½ cup.

Most of the sauces you get from the store contain a lot of salt. You should be extra careful when you buy products like soy sauce, ketchup, relish, BBQ sauce, mustard, and salad dressings.

Last but not least, you should pay more attention to the canned products you purchase such as canned tomatoes or beans. Most of them contain a lot of salt. So limit their usage and read the label before buying them.

Extra Tips That Will Help You With Your Dash Diet

These tips will come in handy and make the transition to the Dash lifestyle a lot easier.

The most important thing to keep in mind is that you need some basic ingredients at hand always. You can buy and stock them for a longer time in your pantry, fridge, or freezer.

Here are some Dash ingredients and products you should always have at hand. This is what your shopping list should look like:

1. whole wheat bread
2. whole wheat flour
3. beans
4. peas
5. carrots
6. broccoli
7. spinach
8. apples
9. oranges
10. bananas
11. rice (wild, brown, white)
12. whole wheat pasta
13. quinoa
14. baking powder
15. low-sodium salad dressings
16. low-sodium tomato sauce
17. tomatoes (canned or not)
18. healthy oils (olive oil, avocado oil, canola oil)
19. fish
20. balsamic vinegar

21. stocks (low-sodium veggie or meat ones)
22. energy bars (granola bars, low-fat ones)
23. whole oats
24. nuts, seeds
25. lemon juice
26. eggs
27. veggies
28. salad greens
29. limes
30. low-fat cheese, yogurt, and natural butter
31. lean meat
32. onions
33. low-sodium soy sauce

Another great tip that will help you commit to your Dash Diet is to get rid of all the products that don't follow the diet's rules. Clean your kitchen and get rid of each product that contains too much sodium.

The Dash Diet is perfect if you want to lose weight in a healthy manner!

The Dash Diet is not really a diet meant to help you lose weight, but once you embrace this healthy lifestyle you will get rid of some pounds.

How is that possible?

Well, it's pretty simple. During the Dash Diet, you only eat 2000 calories per day. This could help you lose weight and achieve your goals.

I've also gathered some easy guidelines to help you get started with your Dash diet:

- Don't start this diet too suddenly. Begin by including at least two servings of veggies and fruits per day and serving only fruits or veggies for dinner. Also, don't switch to whole grains too suddenly. You can start with one whole grain serving per day and move forward from here.
- Don't be afraid to forgive yourself when you slip, and make sure you reward yourself when you reach a certain stage of this diet. When you slip and eat something that's not allowed, you don't have to feel sorry or guilty. Everyone slips and there is a lesson you can learn whenever you make such a dietary mistake. When this happens, just pick up where you left off with your diet and everything will be fine.
- Last but not least, include more physical activity in your lifestyle. Exercising can help lower your blood pressure and help you lose some weight. The combination will be a complete success.

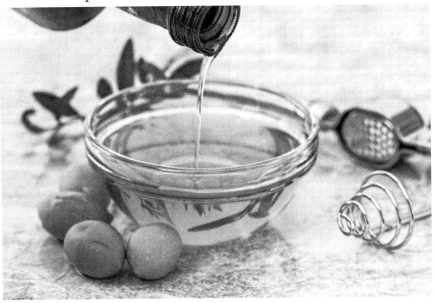

1-Week Meal Plan

Last but not least, here is a 1-week meal plan based on the delicious dishes you'll discover next.

DAY 1

Breakfast: A delicious breakfast frittata + 1 glass low-fat milk

Lunch: A tasty seafood salad

Dinner: A great chicken salad with an amazing peanut dressing

Snacks: 3 lime crackers

Dessert: A fruit soup

DAY 2

Breakfast: A berry muesli + 1 small cup non-fat yogurt

Lunch: A Caesar salad

Dinner: 1 serving balsamic salmon + your favorite side salad

Snacks: 1 potato skin

Dessert: 1 carrot cupcake

DAY 3

Breakfast: 2 spinach pancakes + 1 glass of natural orange juice

Lunch: A chicken sandwich + 1 small side salad

Dinner: 2 baby back ribs + a side salad

Snacks: 1 small cup salsa + 2 carrot sticks

Dessert: 1 small bowl of fruit soup

DAY 4

Breakfast: 2 veggie muffins + 1 glass of low-fat milk

Lunch: 1 serving of Greek chicken salad

Dinner: 2 tuna kabobs + 1 small side salad

Snacks: 2 whole wheat crackers with avocado spread

Dessert: 2 small stuffed peaches

DAY 5

Breakfast: 1 watermelon smoothie

Lunch: 1 bowl chicken soup

Dinner: 2 baked chicken breast halved + 1 side salad

Snacks: Veggie sticks with artichoke dip

Dessert: 1 pineapple bowl

DAY 6

Breakfast: 1 big glass of strawberry and banana smoothie

Lunch: A delicious serving of shrimp soup + 1 small veggie salad

Dinner: 1 delicious bowl of seafood stew

Snacks: 1 serving chickpeas salad + veggie sticks

Dessert: 4 lemon cookies

DAY 7

Breakfast: 1 big cup orange yogurt + 1 spinach pancake

Lunch: 1 big bowl veggie soup

Dinner: 1 serving roasted chicken + 1 side salad

Snacks: 1 cup pistachio dip + some carrot sticks

Dessert: 2 doughnuts + 1 glass natural pineapple juice

Now that you have all the tools you need, it's time to get started with your Dash Diet and your new and amazing lifestyle.

To help you, I prepared a collection of amazing, delicious, and rich Dash Diet recipes that will help you.

So... are you ready for this incredible culinary journey?

Let's get started!

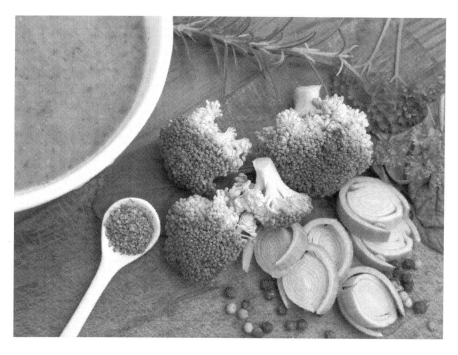

Chapter 2. Dash Diet Recipes for Breakfast

Delicious Berry Muesli

You will really enjoy this amazing breakfast idea!

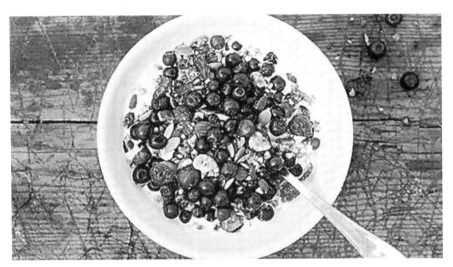

Preparation time: 10 minutes

Cooking time: 0 minutes

Servings: 4

Ingredients:

- 1 cup raw old-fashioned rolled oats
- ½ cup 1% milk
- 1 cup fruit yogurt
- ½ cup mixed raisins, dates and apricots, dried
- ½ cup apple, chopped
- ½ cup blueberries
- ¼ cup walnuts, toasted and chopped

Directions:

1. In a large bowl, mix oats with yogurt, milk, dried fruits, apple and blueberries, toss, divide into bowls, sprinkle walnuts on top and serve.

Enjoy!

Nutrition: calories 121, fat 4, fiber 10, carbs 14, protein 6

Veggie Muffins

You can even take these at the office with you!

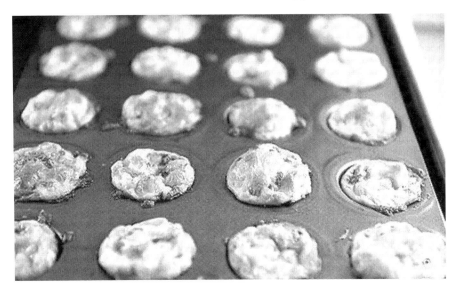

Preparation time: 10 minutes

Cooking time: 40 minutes

Servings: 6

Ingredients:

- 1 cup green onion, chopped
- ¾ cup low-fat cheddar, grated
- 1 cup broccoli, chopped
- 2 cups non-fat milk
- 1 cup tomatoes, chopped
- 1 teaspoon baking powder
- 4 eggs
- Cooking spray
- 1 teaspoon Italian seasoning
- A pinch of black pepper

Directions:

1. Grease a muffin tray with cooking spray and divide broccoli, onion and cheddar in each cup.
2. In a bowl, mix eggs with baking powder, black pepper, Italian seasoning and nonfat milk and whisk well.
3. Divide this into the muffin cups, introduce in the oven and bake at 375 degrees F for 40 minutes.
4. Serve these muffins for breakfast.

Enjoy!

Nutrition: calories 162, fat 6, fiber 6, carbs 12, protein 8

Breakfast Frittata

This is rich, healthy and so delicious!

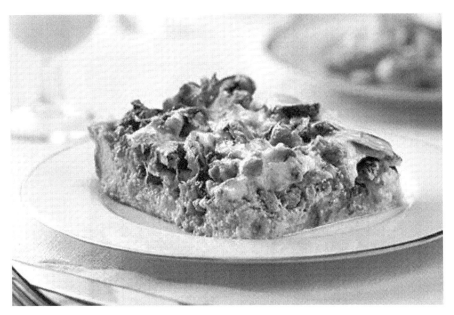

Preparation time: 10 minutes

Cooking time: 1 hour and 10 minutes

Servings: 4

Ingredients:

- 8 ounces whole wheat bread, cubed
- 2 cups non-fat milk
- 12 ounces turkey sausage, chopped
- 1 and ½ cups low-fat cheddar, shredded
- 3 eggs
- ½ cup green onions, chopped
- 1 cup white mushrooms, sliced
- ½ teaspoon sweet paprika
- a pinch of black pepper
- 2 tablespoons low-fat parmesan, grated

Directions:

1. Spread bread cubes on a lined baking sheet, introduce in the oven at 400 degrees F, bake for 8 minutes and leaves aside for now.
2. Meanwhile, heat up a pan over medium-high heat, add sausage, stir, brown for 7 minutes and also leave aside.
3. In a bowl, mix eggs with milk, cheddar, parmesan, pepper and paprika and whisk well.
4. Add sausage, green onions, sausage and mushrooms, toss well and pour everything into a baking dish.
5. Introduce in the oven at 350 degrees F and bake for 50 minutes.
6. Slice, divide between plates and serve for breakfast.

Enjoy!

Nutrition: calories 200, fat 8, fiber 6, carbs 14, protein 12

Delightful Millet Breakfast

This slow-cooked Dash diet breakfast is awesome!

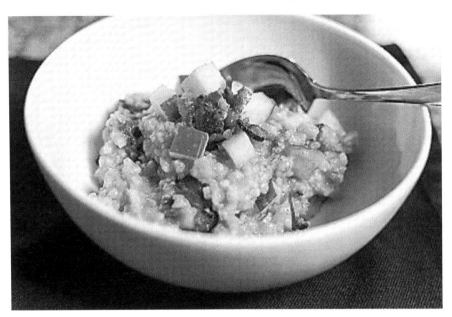

Preparation time: 10 minutes

Cooking time: 2 hours and 30 minutes

Servings: 4

Ingredients:

- 8 bacon strips, cooked and crumbled
- 4 cups water
- 1 cup hulled millet
- 1 cup sweet potato, chopped
- 2 teaspoons ginger, grated
- 1 teaspoon cinnamon powder
- 2 tablespoons stevia
- 1 apple, cored, peeled and chopped

Directions:

1. In your slow cooker, combine millet with water, sweet potato, ginger, cinnamon, stevia and apple, toss, cover and cook on High for 2 hours and 30 minutes.
2. Divide into bowls, sprinkle bacon on top and serve for breakfast.

Enjoy!

Nutrition: calories 172, fat 8, fiber 10, carbs 20, protein 10

Quinoa Bowls

It's the perfect breakfast combination!

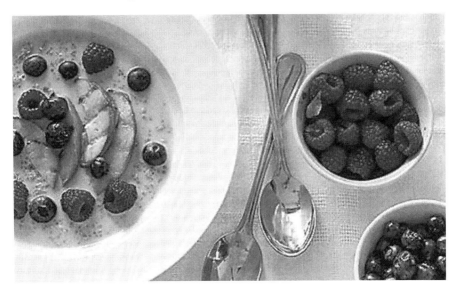

Preparation time: 10 minutes

Cooking time: 23 minutes

Servings: 4

Ingredients:

- 1 peach, cored and sliced
- 1/3 cup quinoa, rinsed
- 1 cup nonfat milk
- ½ teaspoon vanilla extract
- 2 teaspoons stevia
- 12 raspberries
- 12 blueberries

Directions:

1. Heat up a pan with the milk over medium-high heat, add vanilla and stevia, stir and bring to a simmer.
2. Add quinoa, stir, cook for 20 minutes, take off heat and fluff with a fork.
3. Divide quinoa into 2 bowls, top each with peach slices, raspberries and blueberries and serve.

Enjoy!

Nutrition: calories 155, fat 6, fiber 12, carbs 20, protein 8

Watermelon Smoothie

This will give you so much energy, and it will put you in a good mood!

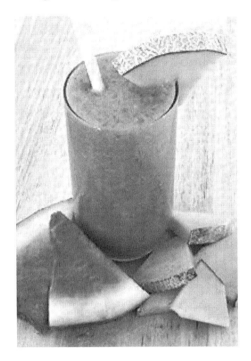

Preparation time: 10 minutes

Cooking time: 0 minutes

Servings: 4

Ingredients:

- 1 cup cantaloupe, chopped
- 1 and ½ cups watermelon, seeded and chopped
- ¼ cup orange juice
- ½ cup non-fat yogurt
- Watermelon wedges for serving

Directions:

1. In your blender, mix yogurt with watermelon and cantaloupe and pulse.
2. Add orange juice, blend again, divide into glasses and serve with watermelon wedges on top.

Enjoy!

Nutrition: calories 140, fat 2, fiber 6, carbs 14, protein 6

Strawberry and Banana Smoothie

This is a 100% Dash diet smoothie!

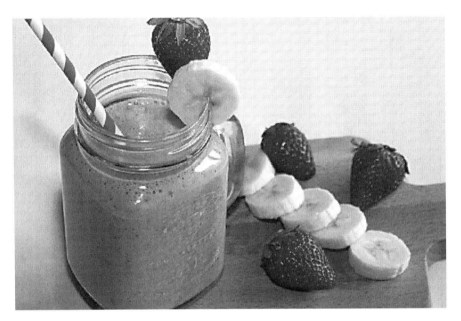

Preparation time: 5 minutes

Cooking time: 0 minutes

Servings: 3

Ingredients:

- 10 strawberries, halved
- ½ teaspoon vanilla extract
- 1 and ½ cups non-fat milk
- 1 tablespoon stevia
- 1 banana, peeled and sliced

Directions:

1. In your blender, mix strawberries with vanilla, milk and banana and pulse well.
2. Divide into glasses and serve right away.

Enjoy!

Nutrition: calories 150, fat 6, fiber 4, carbs 14, protein 8

Shrimp and Artichoke Frittata

You will ask for more once you try it!

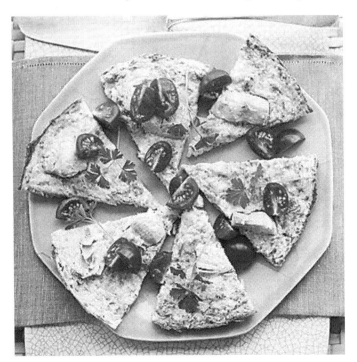

Preparation time: 10 minutes

Cooking time: 10 minutes

Servings: 4

Ingredients:

- 4 ounces shrimp, peeled, deveined and halved
- 3 eggs
- 4 ounces canned artichokes, drained and chopped
- ¼ cup fat-free milk
- A pinch of black pepper
- A pinch of garlic powder
- ¼ cup green onions, chopped

- Cooking spray
- 3 tablespoons low-fat cheddar, grated
- 8 cherry tomatoes, halved
- 1 tablespoon parsley, chopped

Directions:

1. In a bowl, mix eggs with milk, black pepper, garlic powder and green onions and whisk
2. Grease a pan with the cooking spray, heat it up over medium-high heat, add shrimp, stir and cook for 3 minutes.
3. Add eggs mix, spread, reduce heat to medium, cook until the eggs are done and take off heat.
4. Sprinkle artichokes, cheddar cheese, tomatoes and parsley on top, cover pan, leave aside for 4 minutes, divide frittata between plates and serve for breakfast.

Enjoy!

Nutrition: calories 200, fat 4, fiber 6, carbs 10, protein 8

Easy Spinach and Quinoa Pancakes

These are so tasty and so easy to make for breakfast tomorrow!

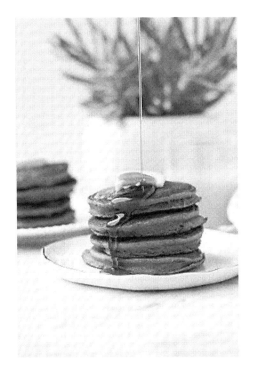

Preparation time: 10 minutes

Cooking time: 30 minutes

Servings: 4

Ingredients:

- 1 and ½ cups water
- 2 garlic cloves, minced
- ¾ cup quinoa
- 2 egg whites
- ½ cup low-fat parmesan, grated
- Black pepper to the taste

- ½ teaspoon basil, dried
- 6 cups baby spinach leaves
- 1 cups salsa
- 4 teaspoons olive oil

Directions:

1. Put the water in a pan, bring to a boil over medium-high heat, add quinoa and the garlic, stir, cover, simmer for 10 minutes, uncover pan, cook for 2 minutes more, take off heat, drain, transfer to a bowl, fluff with a fork and cool down.
2. Add parmesan, basil, black pepper and egg whites and whisk everything well.
3. Heat up a pan with half of the oil over medium heat, make 2 pancakes out of the quinoa mix, place them in the pan, cook for 2 minutes on each side and transfer them to a lined baking sheet.
4. Add the rest of the oil to the pan and also heat up over medium-high heat.
5. Make 2 more quinoa pancakes, cook them for 2 minutes on each side and also transfer them to the baking sheet.
6. Introduce pancakes in the oven at 350 degrees F for 5 minutes and divide them between plates
7. Serve for breakfast.

Enjoy!

Nutrition: calories 170, fat 8, fiber 8, carbs 14, protein 6

Orange Yogurt

This is so delicious and healthy!

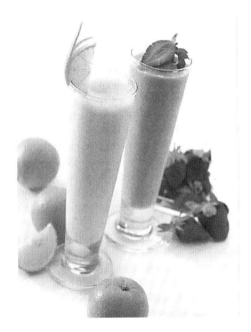

Preparation time: 5 minutes

Cooking time: 0 minutes

Servings: 2

Ingredients:

- 1 cup low-fat milk
- 1 cup orange juice
- 6 ounces low-fat yogurt
- 20 ounces strawberries

Directions:

1. In your blender mix orange juice with milk, yogurt and strawberries and whisk well.

2. Divide into 2 glasses and serve. Enjoy!

Nutrition: calories 100, fat 6, fiber 8, carbs 22, protein 2

Chapter 3. Dash Diet Recipes for Lunch

Easy Shrimp Salad

You only need a few ingredients to make this colored lunch salad!

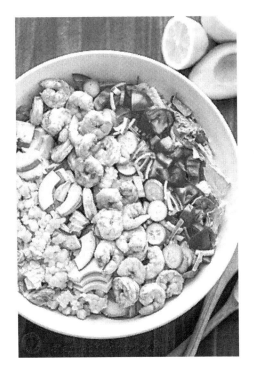

Preparation time: 10 minutes

Cooking time: 20 minutes

Servings: 6

Ingredients:

For the shrimp:

- 2 garlic cloves, minced

- 1 pound shrimp, peeled and deveined
- 1 teaspoon Cajun spice
- 2 tablespoons olive oil

For the salad:

- 6 cups lettuce leaves, torn
- 4 tomatoes, chopped
- 1 small yellow onion, chopped
- 1 cucumber, sliced
- 2 avocados, peeled, pitted and chopped
- 1 cup corn
- Juice of 1 lemon
- ½ bunch parsley, chopped
- 2 tablespoons olive oil
- A pinch of black pepper

Direction:

1. In a bowl, combine the shrimp with Cajun spice and garlic and toss.
2. Heat up a pan with 2 tablespoons oil over medium-high heat, add shrimp, cook for 2 minutes on each side and transfer to a bowl.
3. Add lettuce, tomatoes, onion, cucumber, avocado, corn and a pinch of pepper and toss.
4. In a small bowl, mix 2 tablespoons oil with parsley and lemon juice, whisk well, pour over the salad, toss and serve for lunch.

Enjoy!

Nutrition: calories 210, fat 4, fiber 4, carbs 28, protein 14

Easy Veggie Soup

You will enjoy this simple and delicious soup!

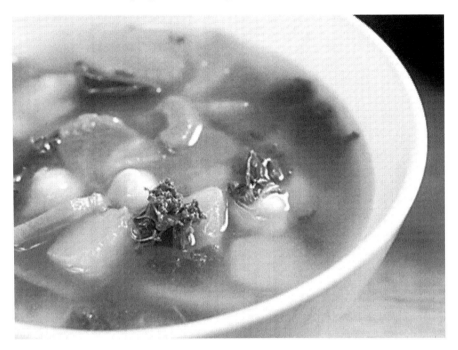

Preparation time: 10 minutes

Cooking time: 20 minutes

Servings: 6

Ingredients:

- 1 tablespoon olive oil
- 1 small yellow onion, chopped
- 2 celery ribs, chopped
- 2 carrots, peeled and chopped
- 2 cups mixed zucchini and cauliflower florets
- A pinch of black pepper
- 1 teaspoon thyme, dried
- ½ teaspoon garlic powder

- 1 teaspoon oregano, dried
- 8 cups low-sodium veggie stock
- 1 bay leaf
- 14 ounces canned tomatoes, low-sodium and chopped

Directions:

1. Heat up a pot with the oil over medium-high heat, add onion, celery and carrots, stir and sauté them for 4 minutes.
2. Add zucchini, cauliflower, black pepper, thyme, garlic powder, oregano, bay leaf, tomatoes and stock, stir, bring to a simmer and cook for 16 minutes.
3. Stir the soup one more time, ladle it into bowls and serve for a dash diet lunch.

Enjoy!

Nutrition: calories 180, fat 2, fiber 8, carbs 28, protein 8

Seafood Salad

This is a very lunch idea!

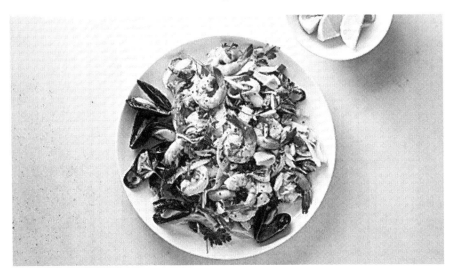

Preparation time: 2 hours and 10 minutes

Cooking time: 1 hour and 30 minutes

Servings: 4

Ingredients:

- 1 big octopus, cleaned
- 1 pound mussels
- 2 pounds clams
- 1 big squid, cut in rings
- 3 garlic cloves, chopped
- 1 celery rib, cut into thirds
- ½ cup celery rib, sliced
- 1 carrot, cut crosswise into 3 pieces
- 1 small white onion, chopped
- 1 bay leaf
- ¾ cup low sodium veggie stock
- 2 cups radicchio, sliced

- 1 red onion, sliced
- 1 cup parsley, chopped
- 1 cup olive oil
- 1 cup red wine vinegar
- Black pepper to the taste

Directions:

1. Place the octopus in a large pot with celery rib cut into thirds, garlic, carrot, bay leaf, white onion and stock. Add water to cover the octopus, cover the pot, bring to a boil over high heat, reduce temperature to low, simmer for 1 hour and 30 minutes. Drain octopus, reserve boiling liquid and leave it aside to cool down.
2. Put ¼ cup octopus cooking liquid in another pot, add mussels, heat up over medium-high heat, cook until they open, transfer to a bowl and leave aside.
3. Add clams to the pan, cover, cook over medium-high heat until they open as well, transfer to the bowl with mussels and leave aside.
4. Add squid to the pan, cover and cook over medium-high heat for 3 minutes, transfer to the bowl with mussels and clams.
5. Meanwhile, slice octopus into small pieces and mix with the rest of the seafood.
6. Add sliced celery, radicchio, red onion, vinegar, olive oil, parsley, salt and pepper, toss and leave aside in the fridge for 2 hours before serving.

Enjoy!

Nutrition: calories 200, fat 8, fiber 8, carbs 28, protein 4

Caesar Salad

It's a very popular salad you can eat even if you are on a Dash diet!

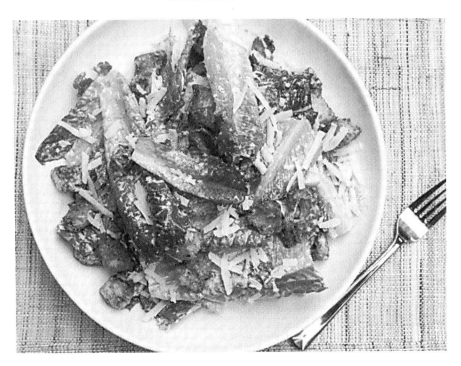

Preparation time: 10 minutes

Cooking time: 12 minutes

Servings: 4

Ingredients:

- 1 pound chicken breast, boneless, skinless and halved
- Cooking spray
- Black pepper to the taste
- ½ cup low-fat feta cheese, cubed
- 2 tablespoons lemon juice
- 1 and ½ teaspoons Dijon mustard
- 1 tablespoon olive oil

- 1 and ½ teaspoons red wine vinegar
- ¾ teaspoon garlic, minced
- 1 tablespoon water
- 1 teaspoon low sodium Worcestershire sauce
- 8 cups lettuce leaves, torn
- 4 tablespoons low-fat parmesan, grated
- 1 and ¼ cups whole wheat croutons

Directions:

1. Spray chicken breasts with some cooking spray and season black pepper to the taste.
2. Heat up your kitchen grill over medium-high heat, add chicken breasts, cook for 6 minutes on each side, transfer to a cutting board, cool down for a few minutes, cut in small pieces, transfer to a salad bowl, add lettuce and croutons and leave aside.
3. In your blender, mix feta with lemon juice, olive oil, mustard, vinegar, Worcestershire sauce and garlic and pulse well.
4. Add the water and half of the parmesan and blend some more.
5. Add this to your salad, toss to coat, sprinkle the rest of the parmesan and serve.

Enjoy!

Nutrition: calories 200, fat 10, fiber 6, carbs 18, protein 10

Greek Chicken Salad

It's Dash diet salad everyone loves!

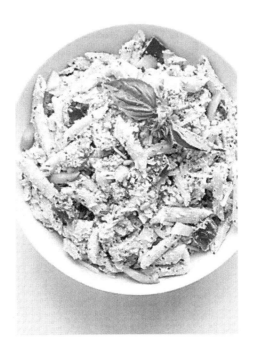

Preparation time: 10 minutes

Cooking time: 0 minutes

Servings: 4

Ingredients:

- 15 ounces canned chickpeas, drained
- 9 ounces chicken breast, already cooked and chopped
- 1 cucumber, chopped
- 4 green onions, chopped
- Black pepper to the taste
- ½ cup fat-free yogurt
- ¼ cup mint, chopped

- 2 cups baby spinach
- 2 garlic cloves, minced
- 1/3 cup low-fat feta cheese, crumbled
- 4 lemon wedges

Directions:

1. In a salad bowl, mix chicken meat with chickpeas, cucumber, onions, mint, garlic, salt and pepper.
2. Add yogurt, spinach and feta and toss to coat.
3. Serve with lemon wedges on the side.

Enjoy!

Nutrition: calories 180, fat 10, fiber 8, carbs 16, protein 10

Chicken Sandwich

It's perfect for a quick lunch!

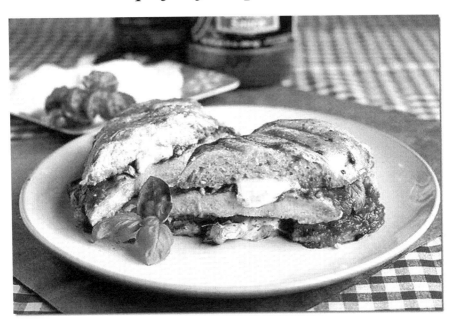

Preparation time: 10 minutes

Cooking time: 10 minutes

Servings: 4

Ingredients:

- 4 chicken breasts
- Cooking spray
- A pinch of Italian seasoning
- 1 eggplant, thinly sliced
- Black pepper to the taste
- A drizzle of olive oil
- ½ cup low-sodium tomato sauce
- 16 basil leaves, torn
- 8 ounces low-fat mozzarella cheese, shredded

- 8 whole wheat bread slices

Directions:

1. Spray chicken with cooking oil, season with black pepper and sprinkle Italian seasoning.
2. Heat up a grill over medium-high heat, add chicken, cook for 5 minutes on each side, transfer to a plate and leave aside for now.
3. Season eggplant slices with black pepper, drizzle olive oil over them, arrange them on preheated grill and cook for a few minute son each side.
4. Arrange 2 bread slices on a working surface, place 1 ounce mozzarella cheese on each bread slice, add 2 eggplant slices on one slice, 1 grilled chicken piece, 2 tablespoon tomato sauce, 4 basil leaves and top with the other bread slice.
5. Repeat this with the rest of the bread slices, making 4 sandwiches.
6. Heat up your Panini press over high heat, add sandwiches, cook them for 4 minutes, leave them to cool down, divide between plates and serve.

Enjoy!

Nutrition: calories 180, fat 4, fiber 12, carbs 28, protein 12

Chicken Soup

It's so flavored and tasty! It's just what you need today!

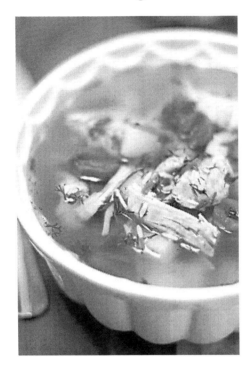

Preparation time: 10 minutes

Cooking time: 2 hours

Servings: 6

Ingredients:

- 1 whole chicken, cut into medium pieces
- 6 celery stalks, chopped
- 6 carrots, sliced
- 1 onion, halved
- A bunch parsley springs
- A bunch dill springs

- 2 tablespoons dill, chopped
- 3 cloves
- 2 tablespoons black peppercorns
- A pinch of black pepper
- 2 bay leaves
- ¼ teaspoon saffron threads

Directions:

1. Put chicken pieces in a pot, add water to cover, bring to a boil over medium-high heat, cook for 15 minutes and skim foam.
2. Add celery, onion, carrots, parsley springs, dill springs, whole cloves, bay leaves, peppercorns and some black pepper, stir, cover pot, reduce heat to medium-low and simmer for 1 hour and 30 minutes.
3. Take chicken pieces out and leave them aside to cool down.
4. Strain soup into another pot, reserve carrots and celery but discard herbs and spices.
5. Discard bones from the chicken, cut meat into strips and return to pot.
6. Heat up the soup with reserved veggies, add chicken pieces, crushed saffron and chopped dill and stir.
7. Ladle soup into bowls and serve.

Enjoy!

Nutrition: calories 200, fat 10, fiber 4, carbs 16, protein 12

Pumpkin Soup

It's easy to make, rich and delicious!

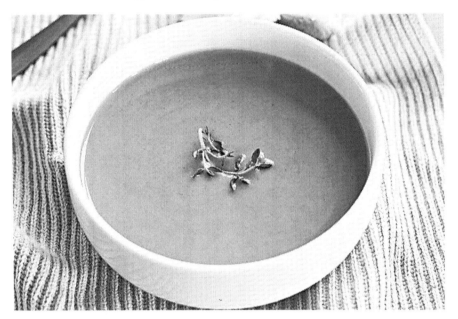

Preparation time: 10 minutes

Cooking time: 10 minutes

Servings: 4

Ingredients:

- 1 yellow onion, chopped
- ¾ cup water
- 15 ounces pumpkin puree
- 2 cups low-sodium veggie stock
- ½ teaspoon cinnamon powder
- ¼ teaspoon nutmeg, ground
- 1 cup fat-free milk
- A pinch of black pepper
- 1 green onion, chopped

Directions:

1. Put the water in a pot, bring to a simmer over medium heat, add onion, stock and pumpkin puree and stir.
2. Add cinnamon, nutmeg, milk and black pepper, stir, cook for 10 minutes, ladle into bowls, sprinkle green onion on top and serve.

Enjoy!

Nutrition: calories 180, fat 10, fiber 10, carbs 22, protein 14

Spicy Black Bean Soup

This is a special Dash diet soup!

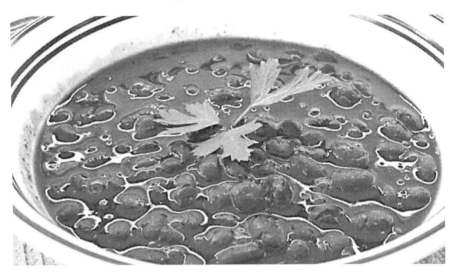

Preparation time: 10 minutes

Cooking time: 1 hour and 45 minutes

Servings: 8

Ingredients:

- 1 pound black beans, soaked overnight and drained
- 2 yellow onions, chopped
- 2 quarts low-sodium veggie stock
- 2 tablespoons olive oil
- 6 garlic cloves, minced
- 2 tomatoes, chopped
- 2 jalapenos, chopped
- ½ teaspoon oregano, dried
- 1 teaspoon cumin, ground
- 1 teaspoon ginger, grated
- 2 bay leaves
- 1 tablespoon chili powder

- 3 tablespoons balsamic vinegar
- Black pepper to the taste
- ½ cup scallions, chopped

Directions:

1. Put the stock in a pot, bring to a simmer over medium heat, add beans, cover and cook for 45 minutes.
2. Meanwhile, heat up a pan with the oil over medium-high heat, add ginger, garlic and onion, stir and cook for 5 minutes.
3. Add tomatoes, cumin, jalapeno, oregano and chili powder, stir, cook for 3 minutes more and transfer to the pot with the beans.
4. Add bay leaves, cover the pot and cook the soup for 40 minutes more.
5. Add vinegar, stir, cook the soup for 15 minutes more, discard bay leaves, blend the soup using an immersion blender, ladle into bowls and serve with scallions on top.

Enjoy!

Nutrition: calories 220, fat 10, fiber 10, carbs 34, protein 14

Shrimp Soup

Enjoy this amazing soup as soon as possible!

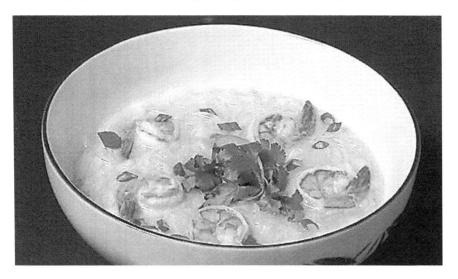

Preparation time: 10 minutes

Cooking time: 25 minutes

Servings: 6

Ingredients:

- 8 ounces shrimp, peeled and deveined
- 1 stalk lemongrass, crushed
- 2 small ginger pieces, grated
- 6 cup low-sodium chicken stock
- 2 jalapenos, chopped
- 4 lime leaves
- 1 and ½ cups pineapple, chopped
- 1 cup shiitake mushroom caps, chopped
- 1 tomato, chopped
- ½ bell pepper, cubed
- 1 teaspoon stevia
- ¼ cup lime juice

- 1/3 cup cilantro, chopped
- 2 scallions, sliced

Directions:

1. In a pot, mix ginger with lemongrass, stock, jalapenos and lime leaves, stir, bring to a boil over medium heat, cover, cook for 15 minutes, strain liquid in a bowl and discard solids.
2. Return soup to the pot again, add pineapple, tomato, mushrooms, bell pepper, sugar and fish sauce, stir, bring to a boil over medium heat, cook for 5 minutes, add shrimp and cook for 3 more minutes.
3. Add lime juice, cilantro and scallions, stir, ladle into soup bowls and serve.

Enjoy!

Nutrition: calories 190, fat 8, fiber 6, carbs 30, protein 6

Chapter 4. Dash Diet Recipes for Dinner

Seafood Stew

This is a simple recipe you can prepare for dinner!

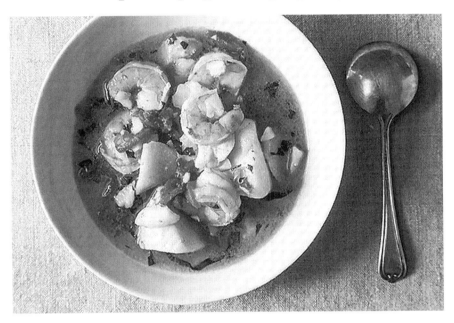

Preparation time: 10 minutes

Cooking time: 12 minutes

Servings: 4

Ingredients:

- 12 jumbo shrimp, peeled (shells reserved) and deveined
- 4 parsley springs
- ¼ cup parsley, chopped
- 1 garlic clove, minced
- 1 tablespoon garlic, minced

- 1 tablespoon extra virgin olive oil
- ¼ cup shallot, chopped
- 1 cup low sodium veggie stock
- 2 dozen clams, scrubbed
- 1 pound mussels, scrubbed
- Black pepper to the taste
- 1 tomato, chopped
- 8 scallops, halved horizontally
- 2 cups water

Directions:

1. Heat up a pan over high heat, add shrimp shells and 1 garlic clove, stir and cook for 2 minutes.
2. Add parsley springs and water, stir, bring to a boil, cook for 3 minutes, strain into a bowl and leave aside for now.
3. Meanwhile, heat up another pan with the olive oil over medium-high heat, add 1 tablespoon garlic and shallots, stir and cook for 1 minute.
4. Add veggie and shrimp stock, clams and mussels, bring to a simmer and cook for 4 minutes.
5. Divide clams and mussels into bowls, sprinkle chopped parsley and leave aside.
6. Season broth with black pepper, add scallops, shrimp and tomato, cover and cook for 2 more minutes over medium heat.
7. Add this mix to the bowls, sprinkle chopped parsley and serve.

Enjoy!

Nutrition: calories 180, fat 4, fiber 6, carbs 14, protein 6

Tuna Kabobs

They taste divine!

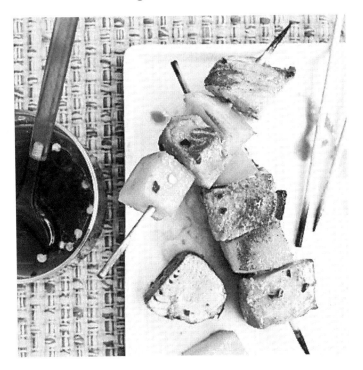

Preparation time: 30 minutes

Cooking time: 10 minutes

Servings: 16

Ingredients:

- ¼ cup low-sodium soy sauce
- 1 pound tuna steaks, cubed in 16 pieces
- 2 tablespoons rice vinegar
- Black pepper to the taste
- 1 tablespoon sesame seeds
- 2 tablespoons canola oil
- 16 pieces pickled ginger

Directions:

1. In a bowl, mix soy sauce with vinegar and tuna, toss to coat, cover bowl and keep in the fridge for 30 minutes.
2. Discard marinade, pat dry tuna and sprinkle with black pepper and sesame seeds.
3. Heat up a pan with the oil over medium heat, add tuna pieces, cook them until they are pink in the center and brown on the outside, take off heat and transfer them to a plate.
4. Thread ginger and tuna cubes on the skewers, arrange the kabobs on a platter and serve them with a side salad.

Enjoy!

Nutrition: calories 180, fat 10, fiber 8, carbs 24, protein 8

Balsamic Salmon

This will make your evening a success!

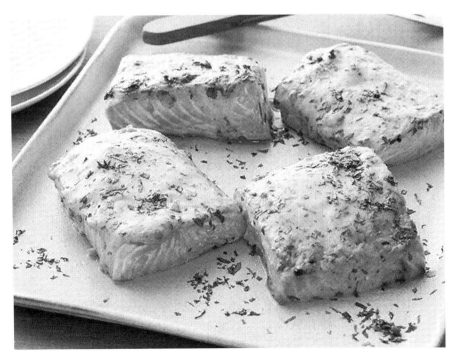

Preparation time: 10 minutes

Cooking time: 35 minutes

Servings: 6

Ingredients:

- 2 pounds salmon fillets, boneless and skin on
- 1 garlic clove, minced
- ¼ cup real maple syrup
- ¼ cup balsamic vinegar
- A pinch of black pepper
- 1 tablespoon mint, chopped
- Cooking spray

Directions:

1. Heat up a pan over medium-low heat, add maple syrup, vinegar and garlic, whisk, heat up for 1 minutes, transfer this to a bowl and leave aside to cool down.
2. Spray a baking sheet with cooking spray, add salmon fillets, season them with black pepper and brush with half of the maple glaze.
3. Introduce in the oven at 450 degrees F, bake for 10 minutes, brush salmon with the rest of the glaze and bake for 20 minutes more.
4. Divide between plates, sprinkle mint on top and serve.

Enjoy!

Nutrition: calories 210, fat 8, fiber 8, carbs 20, protein 8

Baked Chicken Breasts

This is so flavored and rich!

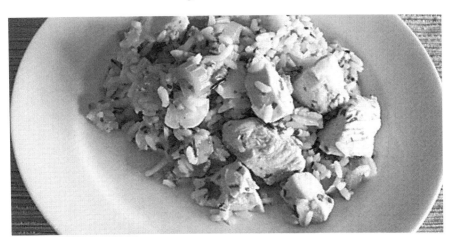

Preparation time: 40 minutes

Cooking time: 1 hour and 10 minutes

Servings: 6

Ingredients:

- 1 and ½ cups celery, chopped
- 1 pound chicken breast halves, skinless, boneless and cut into medium pieces
- 1 and ½ cups pearl onions
- 2 cups chicken stock
- 1 teaspoon tarragon, chopped
- ¾ cup white rice
- 1 and ½ cups white wine
- ¾ cup wild rice

Directions:

1. Put half of the stock in a pot, add chicken, tarragon, onions and celery, stir, bring to a simmer over medium heat, cook for 10 minutes, take off heat and leave aside to cool down.
2. In a baking dish, mix the rest of the stock with white and wild rice, stir and leave aside for 30 minutes.
3. Add chicken and the veggies, cover, introduce in the oven at 300 degrees F and bake for 1 hour.
4. Divide between plates and serve right away.

Enjoy!

Nutrition: calories 300, fat 2, fiber 4, carbs 28, protein 36

Roasted Chicken

This roasted chicken is simply incredible!

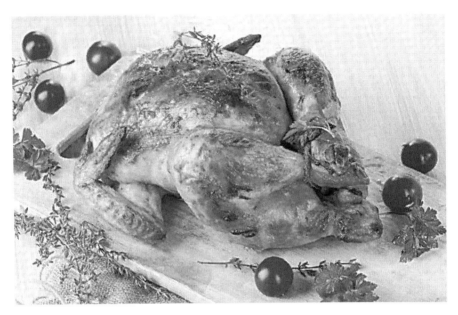

Preparation time: 10 minutes

Cooking time: 1 hour and 30 minutes

Servings: 8

Ingredients:

- 1 whole chicken
- 1 garlic clove, minced
- 1 tablespoon rosemary, chopped
- 1 tablespoon olive oil
- Black pepper to the taste
- ½ cup balsamic vinegar
- 1 teaspoon stevia
- 8 rosemary springs

Directions:

1. In a bowl, mix garlic with rosemary and stir.
2. Rub chicken with black pepper, the oil and rosemary mix, put it in a roasting pan, introduce in the oven at 350 degrees F and roast for 1 hour and 20 minutes basting with pan juices from time to time.
3. Meanwhile, heat up a pan with the vinegar over medium heat, add stevia, stir and cook until it dissolves.
4. Carve the chicken, divide it between plates and serve with the vinegar mix drizzled all over.

Enjoy!

Nutrition: calories 345, fat 10, fiber 2, carbs 20, protein 44

Chicken Salad and Peanut Dressing

I warmly recommend you to try this Dash diet salad for dinner!

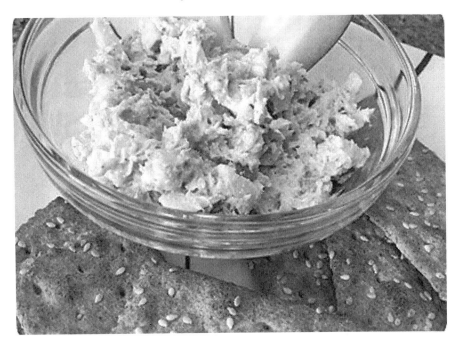

Preparation time: 10 minutes

Cooking time: 0 minutes

Servings: 6

Ingredients:

- 4 cups chicken, cooked, boneless, skinless and shredded
- ¼ cup olive oil
- 1/3 cup rice wine vinegar
- 2 teaspoons sesame oil
- ¼ cup low-sodium peanut sauce
- ½ napa cabbage head, shredded
- 1 cup carrot, grated

- 6 scallions, sliced
- Black pepper to the taste
- 2 teaspoons sesame seeds

Directions:

1. In a bowl, mix olive oil with peanut sauce, vinegar and sesame oil and whisk very well.
2. In a salad bowl, mix chicken with 4 scallions, cabbage and carrot.
3. Add peanut dressing and pepper and toss to coat.
4. Divide between plates, sprinkle sesame seeds and the rest of the scallions on top and serve.

Enjoy!

Nutrition: calories 200, fat 4, fiber 4, carbs 16, protein 12

Braised Brisket

Get all the ingredients you need and make this brisket today!

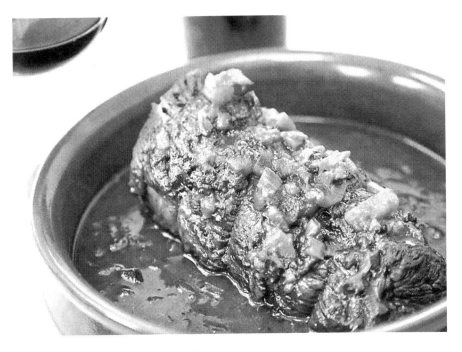

Preparation time: 10 minutes

Cooking time: 7 hours and 15 minutes

Servings: 6

Ingredients:

- 1 pound sweet onion, chopped
- 4 pounds beef brisket
- 1 pound carrot, chopped
- 8 earl grey tea bags
- ½ pound celery, chopped
- A pinch of salt
- Black pepper to the taste
- 4 cups water

For the sauce:

- 16 ounces canned tomatoes, chopped
- ½ pound celery, chopped
- 1 ounce of garlic, minced
- 4 ounces olive oil
- 1 pound sweet onion, chopped
- 8 earl grey tea bags
- 1 tablespoon stevia
- 1 cup white vinegar

Directions:

1. Put the water in a pot, add 1 pound onion, 1 pound carrot, ½ pound celery, salt and pepper, stir and bring to a simmer over medium-high heat.
2. Add beef brisket and 8 tea bags, stir, cover, reduce heat to medium-low and cook for 7 hours.
3. Meanwhile, heat up a pan with the oil over medium-high heat, add 1 pound onion, stir and sauté for 10 minutes.
4. Add garlic, ½ pound celery, tomatoes, stevia, vinegar and 8 tea bags, stir, bring to a simmer, cook until veggies are done and discard tea bags at the end.
5. Transfer beef brisket to a cutting board, leave aside to cool down, slice, divide between plates and serve with the sauce drizzled all over.

Enjoy!

Nutrition: calories 400, fat 14, fiber 8, carbs 36, protein 6

Veggie Stir Fry

It's a light Dash diet dinner option!

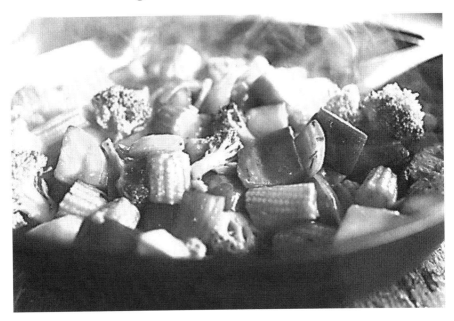

Preparation time: 10 minutes

Cooking time: 6 minutes

Servings: 8

Ingredients:

- 2 tablespoons low-sodium veggie stock
- ½ cup low-sodium soy sauce
- 2 tablespoons cornstarch
- 2 tablespoons stevia
- 1 tablespoon ginger, grated
- 1 yellow onion, chopped
- 2 tablespoons olive oil
- 1 red bell pepper, cut into medium wedges
- 1 yellow bell pepper, cut into medium wedges
- 2 garlic cloves, minced

- 2 zucchinis, cut into medium wedges
- 13 ounces baby corn, halved
- 1 small broccoli head, florets separated

Directions:

1. In a bowl, mix the stock with the soy sauce, cornstarch, stevia and ginger and whisk well.
2. Heat up a pan with the oil over medium-high heat, add the onion, stir and cook for 1-2 minutes.
3. Add red bell pepper, yellow bell pepper, garlic, zucchini, corn, broccoli and the cornstarch mix, stir, cook for 8 minutes, divide into bowls and serve.

Enjoy!

Nutrition: calories 172, fat 8, fiber 10, carbs 22, protein 10

Mexican Quinoa Mix

Everyone will like this delicious mix!

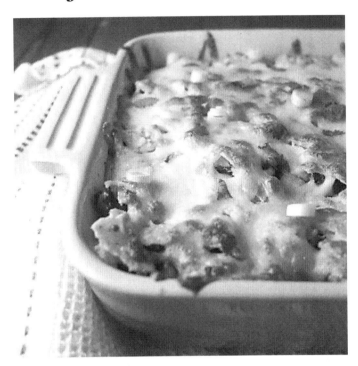

Preparation time: 10 minutes

Cooking time: 40 minutes

Servings: 4

Ingredients:

- 1 cup quinoa, dry
- 2 cups low-sodium veggie stock
- 1 tablespoon olive oil
- 2 red onions, chopped
- 2 garlic cloves, minced
- 2 red bell peppers, chopped
- 1 pound chicken meat, ground

- 2 cups low-sodium tomato sauce
- 1 cup canned kidney beans, drained and no-salt-added
- 2 ounces low-fat cheese, grated

Directions:

1. Put the stock in a pot, add quinoa, bring to a simmer over medium heat, cook for 15 minutes and take off heat.
2. Heat up a pan with the oil over medium-high heat, add onions and garlic, stir and cook for 2-4 minutes.
3. Add bell pepper, chicken and quinoa and toss a bit.
4. Add tomato sauce and kidney beans and toss again.
5. Sprinkle the cheese all over, introduce the pan in the oven and cook at 360 degrees F for 20 minutes.
6. Slice, divide between plates and serve.

Enjoy!

Nutrition: calories 240, fat 20, fiber 4, carbs 20, protein 38

Baby Back Ribs

It's a fulfilling Dash diet dinner idea!

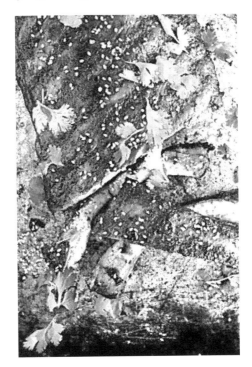

Preparation time: 1 hour and 10 minutes

Cooking time: 1 hour

Servings: 6

Ingredients:

- 12 green tea bags, strings removed
- Salt and black pepper to the taste
- 26 pork back ribs
- 1 onion, julienned
- 3 carrots, chopped
- 6 celery ribs, chopped
- 1 Jicama, roughly chopped

- 2 green apples, chopped
- 4 scallions, chopped
- ½ cup rice wine vinegar
- 1 green tea and lemon tea bag
- 1 cup olive oil

Directions:

1. In a pot, mix ribs with salt, pepper, half of the carrot, onion, half of the celery and 8 tea bags, stir, bring to a simmer over medium heat, cover and cook for 1 hour.
2. Meanwhile, in a bowl, mix vinegar with green tea and lemon tea bag, stir, leave aside for 1 hour and discard tea bags.
3. In a bowl, mix apple with the rest of the celery ribs, the rest of the carrot, Jicama, scallions and oil and toss to coat.
4. Add vinaigrette and toss to coat.
5. Divide ribs between plates, return the cooking liquid to medium heat, bring to a simmer, add the rest of the tea bags, cook for 10 minutes and discard them.
6. Drizzle this over ribs and serve with the salad on the side.

Enjoy!

Nutrition: calories 400, fat 14, fiber 6, carbs 40, protein 8

Chapter 5. Dash Diet Dessert Recipes

Carrot Cupcakes

I just love these Dash diet cupcakes!

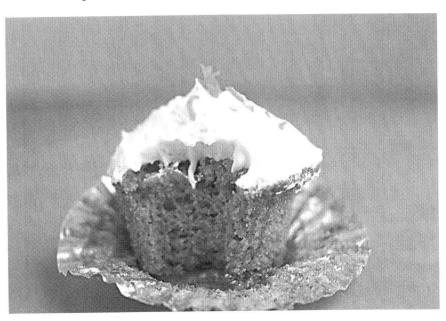

Preparation time: 1 hour and 10 minutes

Cooking time: 0 minutes

Servings: 6

Ingredients:

- 1 cup almonds
- 2 cups carrot pulp
- 1 cup dates, chopped
- ½ teaspoon ginger, grated
- 1 teaspoon cinnamon powder
- A pinch of nutmeg

- ¾ cup raisins

for the frosting:

- 1 cup cashews, soaked for 1 hour and drained
- A splash of water
- 1 teaspoon lemon juice
- 6 dates, pitted, soaked for 1 hour and drained

Directions:

1. In your food processor, mix 1 cup walnuts with 1 cup dates, carrot pulp, 1 teaspoon cinnamon, ginger, a pinch of nutmeg and the raisins, blend and divide this into cupcake cups.
2. Clean your food processor, add 1 cup cashews, 6 dates, a splash of water and the lemon juice and blend these as well.
3. Divide the frosting on the cupcakes, introduce them in the fridge for 1 hour and serve.

Enjoy!

Nutrition: calories 150, fat 4, fiber 4, carbs 16, protein 8

Dash Diet Doughnuts

Did you ever imagine you could have doughnuts if you are on a diet?

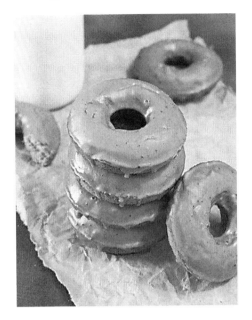

Preparation time: 10 minutes

Cooking time: 10 minutes

Servings: 8

Ingredients:

- 3 tablespoons stevia
- 1 cup whole wheat flour
- 1 teaspoon baking powder
- 2 tablespoons matcha powder
- ½ teaspoon vanilla extract
- ½ cup low-fat buttermilk
- 1 egg, whisked
- 1 tablespoon avocado oil
- Cooking spray

Directions:

1. In a bowl, mix flour with matcha powder, stevia and baking powder and whisk.
2. Add buttermilk, vanilla extract, egg and oil and stir using your mixer.
3. Divide into doughnut cavities after you've sprayed with cooking oil, introduce in the oven at 400 degrees F and bake for 10 minutes.
4. Serve them cold.

Enjoy!

Nutrition: calories 200, fat 4, fiber 6, carbs 26, protein 12

Sweet Seeds Bars

These are so tasty!

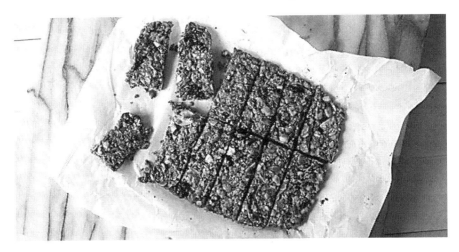

Preparation time: 10 minutes

Cooking time: 30 minutes

Servings: 6

Ingredients:

- 1 pound sunflower seeds, walnuts, almonds and peanuts, chopped
- 2 cups honey
- 6 tablespoons stevia

Directions:

1. Spread nuts on a baking sheet, introduce in the oven at 350 degrees F and roast them for 10 minutes.
2. Meanwhile, in a pan, mix honey with stevia, stir and bring to a boil over medium heat.

3. Take nuts out of the oven, add them to the pan, stir and cook for 15 minutes more.
4. Pour this mix into a pan brushed with water, spread evenly and leave aside to cool down.
5. Turn pan upside down, cut rectangles and serve them cold.

Enjoy!

Nutrition: calories 140, fat 4, fiber 3, carbs 14, protein 8

Berries and Orange Sauce

It's such a sweet Dash diet delight!

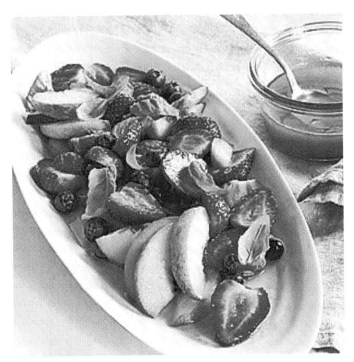

Preparation time: 10 minutes

Cooking time: 15 minutes

Servings: 4

Ingredients:

- 1 cup orange juice
- 1 and ½ tablespoons stevia
- 1 and ½ tablespoons champagne vinegar
- 1 tablespoon olive oil
- 1 pound strawberries, halved
- 1 and ½ cups blueberries
- 1 peach, roughly chopped

- ¼ cup basil leaves, torn

Directions:

1. In a pot, mix orange juice with stevia and vinegar, stir, bring to a boil over medium-high heat, simmer for 15 minutes, add oil, stir, take off heat and leave aside for a couple of minutes.
2. In a bowl, mix blueberries with strawberries and peach wedges, add orange vinaigrettes, toss to coat, sprinkle basil on top and serve!

Enjoy!

Nutrition: calories 100, fat 2, fiber 6, carbs 20, protein 4

Grapefruit Granita

It's such a fresh dessert!

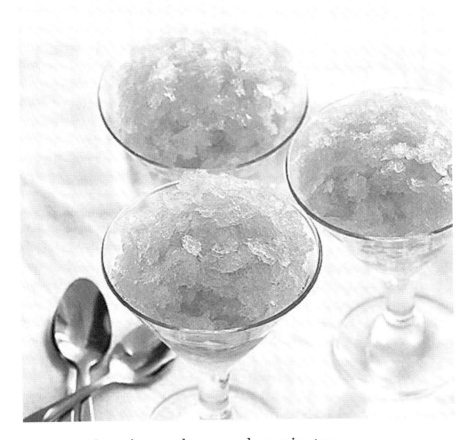

Preparation time: 4 hours and 20 minutes

Cooking time: 3 minutes

Servings: 3

Ingredients:

- 1 cup water
- 1 cup coconut sugar
- ½ cup mint, chopped

- 64 ounces red grapefruit juice

Directions:

1. Put the water in a pan, bring to a boil over medium heat, add sugar, stir until it dissolves, take off heat, add mint, stir, cover and leave aside for 5 minutes
2. Strain into a container, add grapefruit juice, stir, cover and freeze for 4 hours before serving

Enjoy!

Nutrition: calories 80, fat 0, fiber 0, carbs 14, protein 3

Stewed Plums

It's the sweetest stew ever!

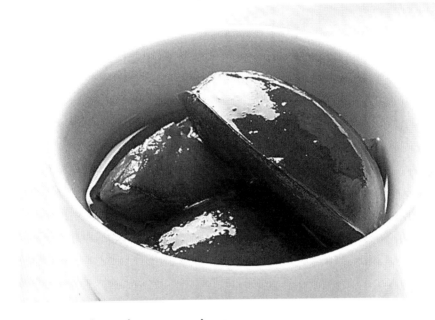

Preparation time: 10 minutes

Cooking time: 15 minutes

Servings: 4

Ingredients:

- 16 plums, stoned and halved
- 1 cup water
- ½ cup coconut sugar
- 5 cardamom pods, crushed

Directions:

1. Put water in a pot, add sugar, heat up over medium-low heat, add cardamom, bring to a boil and simmer for 10 minutes.
2. Add plums, stir gently, cover pot and cook for 5 minutes.
3. Leave plums aside to cool down before serving.

Enjoy!

Nutrition: calories 110, fat 2, fiber 4, carbs 12, protein 6

Lemon Cookies

These cookies taste special!

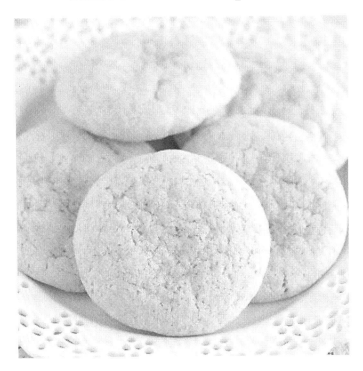

Preparation time: 2 hours and 10 minutes

Cooking time: 0 minutes

Servings: 10

Ingredients:

- 1/3 cup cashew butter
- 1 and ½ tablespoons coconut oil
- 2 tablespoons coconut butter
- 5 tablespoons lemon juice
- ½ teaspoon lemon zest, grated
- 1 tablespoons maple syrup

Directions:

1. In a bowl, mix cashew butter with coconut one, coconut oil, lemon juice, lemon zest and maple syrup and stir until you obtain a creamy mix.
2. Line a tray with parchment paper, scoop 1 tablespoon of lemon cookie mix on the tray, repeat with the rest of the dough and freeze for 2 hours before serving.

Enjoy!

Nutrition: calories 121, fat 2, fiber 8, carbs 18, protein 2

Pineapple Bowls

Your day just got better with this dessert!

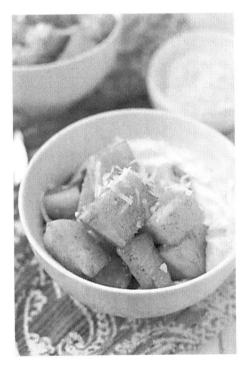

Preparation time: 10 minutes

Cooking time: 0 minutes

Servings: 6

Ingredients:

- 4 cups pineapple pieces
- 2 tablespoons honey
- ½ cup whole wheat and barley cereals
- 12 ounces low-fat vanilla yogurt
- ¼ cup coconut, toasted and shredded

Directions:

1. Divide pineapple pieces into 6 bowls, add yogurt and toss
2. Sprinkle cereals and toasted coconut on top and serve right away.

Enjoy!

Nutrition: calories 130, fat 6, fiber 6, carbs 12, protein 6

Stuffed Peaches

This dessert will really impress you!

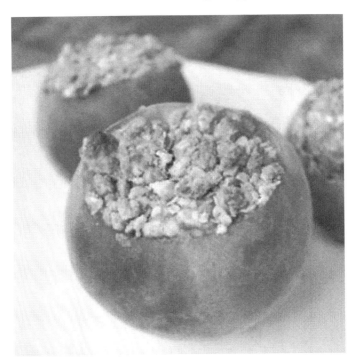

Preparation time: 10 minutes

Cooking time: 40 minutes

Servings: 4

Ingredients:

- ½ cup favorite dried fruits
- ¼ cup almonds, toasted
- 4 peaches, pitted and tops cut off
- 2 tablespoons graham crackers, crumbled
- ¼ teaspoon allspice, ground
- 2 tablespoons stevia
- ½ cup fat-free yogurt

- 12 ounces canned peach nectar

Directions:

1. Scoop each peach, chop the pulp, put into a bowl, add dried fruits and mix.
2. Also add almonds, crackers, sugar and allspice and stir everything.
3. Stuff each peach with this mix, place them on a baking sheet, drizzle the nectar all over, introduce in the oven at 350 degrees F and bake for 40 minutes.
4. Divide peaches on plates, drizzle pan juices, top with yogurt and serve.

Enjoy!

Nutrition: calories 130, fat 2, fiber 6, carbs 14, protein 10

Fruit Soup

Have you ever tried such soup?

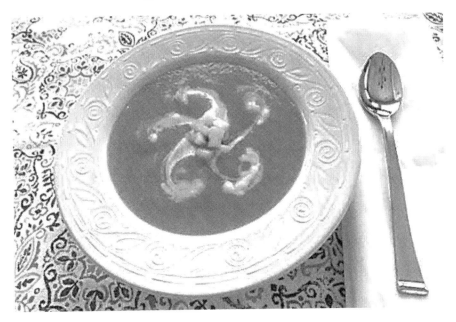

Preparation time: 1 hour and 10 minutes

Cooking time: 0 minutes

Servings: 4

Ingredients:

- 2 cups cantaloupe, cut into medium pieces
- 1 and ½ cups canned peach nectar
- 6 ounces peach, pitted, peeled and cut into medium pieces
- 2 tablespoons lemon juice
- 1 cup raspberries
- A few mint leaves, torn

Directions:

1. In your blender, mix cantaloupe with peach nectar, peach and lemon juice and pulse well.
2. Transfer to a bowl, cover and keep in the fridge for 1 hour.
3. Divide this into bowl, top with raspberries and mint leaves and serve,

Enjoy!

Nutrition: calories 140, fat 2, fiber 2, carbs 16, protein 6

Chapter 6. Dash Diet Snack and Appetizer Recipes

Artichoke Dip

This great party dip will impress your guests!

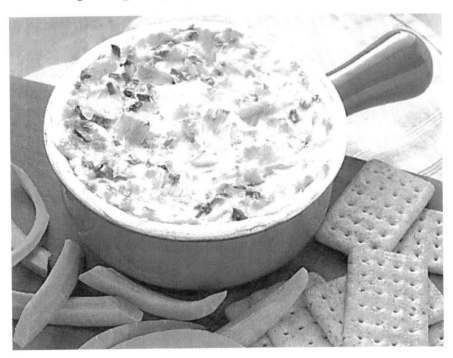

Preparation time: 10 minutes

Cooking time: 30 minutes

Servings: 8

Ingredients:

- 4 cups spinach, chopped
- 2 cups artichoke hearts
- Black pepper to the taste
- 1 teaspoon thyme, chopped

- 2 garlic cloves, minced
- 1 cup canned white beans, drained and rinsed
- 1 tablespoon parsley, chopped
- 2 tablespoons low-fat parmesan, grated
- ½ cup low-fat sour cream

Directions:

1. In a baking dish, mix artichokes with spinach, black pepper, thyme, garlic, beans, parsley, parmesan and sour cream, stir well, introduce in the oven at 350 degrees F and bake for 30 minutes.
2. Mash using a potato masher, divide into bowls and serve.

Enjoy!

Nutrition: calories 181, fat 4, fiber 6, carbs 26, protein 8

Avocado Spread

This delicious spread is simply incredible!

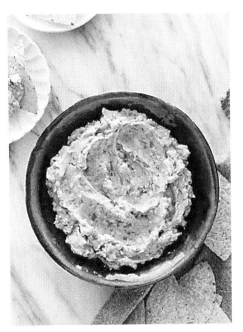

Preparation time: 10 minutes

Cooking time: 0 minutes

Servings: 4

Ingredients:

- 2 teaspoons yellow onion, chopped
- 1 avocado, peeled, pitted and mashed with a fork
- ½ cup fat-free sour cream
- A splash of hot sauce

Directions:

1. In a bowl, mix sour cream with onion, avocado and hot sauce, whisk well and serve right away.

Enjoy!

Nutrition: calories 139, fat 2, fiber 4, carbs 14, protein 10

Potato Skins

It's a simple Dash diet appetizer!

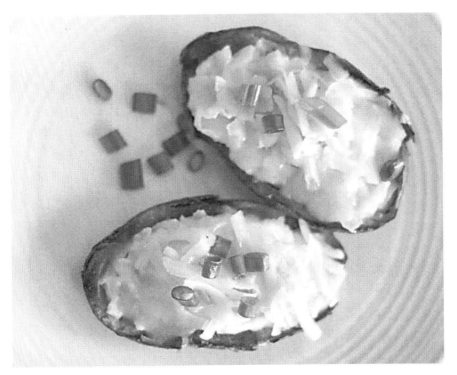

Preparation time: 10 minutes

Cooking time: 1 hour and 10 minutes

Servings: 2

Ingredients:

- Cooking spray
- 2 potatoes
- 1 tablespoon spring onion, chopped
- 1 tablespoon rosemary, chopped
- A pinch of black pepper

Directions:

1. Prick potatoes with a fork, place them on a baking sheet, introduce in the oven at 375 degrees F and bake for 1 hour.
2. Cut potatoes into halves and scoop almost all the flesh.
3. Spray potato skins with cooking spray, sprinkle black pepper, spring onions and rosemary, introduce them in the oven again and bake for 10 minutes.
4. Divide potato skins between plates and serve.

Enjoy!

Nutrition: calories 200, fat 8, fiber 8, carbs 22, protein 4

Classic Salsa

It's a dash diet salsa full of intense colors and tastes!

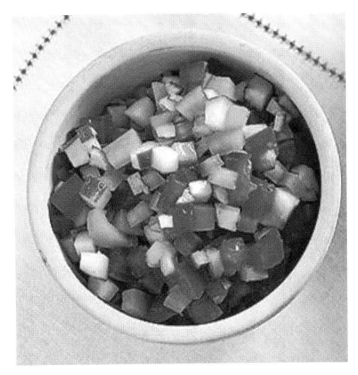

Preparation time: 10 minutes

Cooking time: 0 minutes

Servings: 6

Ingredients:

- 2 tomatoes, chopped
- 1 cucumber, chopped
- 1 yellow bell pepper, chopped
- 1 small red onion, chopped
- Salt and black pepper to the taste
- 1 tablespoon extra virgin olive oil
- 1 tablespoon red wine vinegar

Directions:

1. In a bowl, mix tomatoes with cucumber, onion and bell pepper and stir.
2. Add salt, pepper to the taste, vinegar and oil, toss to coat and serve right away.

Enjoy!

Nutrition: calories 123, fat 4, fiber 4, carbs 16, protein 6

Chickpeas Salsa

Find out how to make the best salsa!

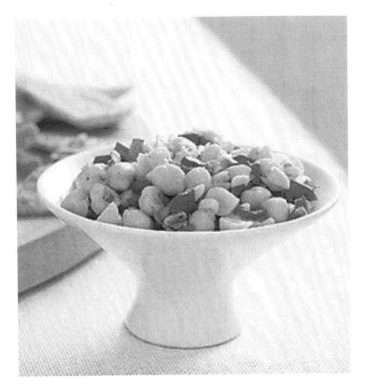

Preparation time: 10 minutes

Cooking time: 0 minutes

Servings: 6

Ingredients:

- 4 scallions, sliced
- 1 cup arugula, chopped
- 15 ounces canned chickpeas, roughly chopped
- Salt and black pepper to the taste
- 2 jarred red peppers, roasted and chopped
- 2 tablespoons extra virgin olive oil

- 2 tablespoons lemon juice

Directions:

1. In a bowl, mix chickpeas with arugula, scallions, red peppers, salt, pepper, lemon juice and olive oil and stir very well.
2. Divide into small bowls and serve.

Enjoy!

Nutrition: calories 155, fat 8, fiber 5, carbs 18, protein 8

Pomegranate Dip

The taste is divine!

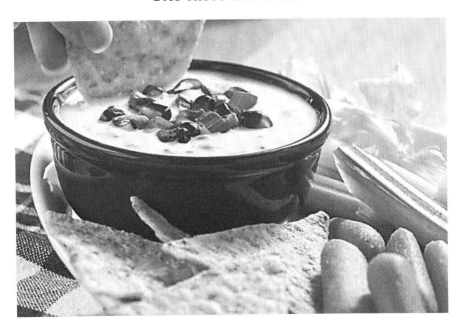

Preparation time: 1 hour and 10 minutes

Cooking time: 0 minutes

Servings: 8

Ingredients:

- ½ cup pomegranate seeds+ some more for serving
- 1 cup fat-free yogurt
- 1 tablespoon cilantro, chopped
- 1 scallion, sliced
- 1 cup low-fat sour cream
- 1 garlic clove, minced
- Black pepper to the taste
- ½ teaspoon lemon juice

Directions:

1. In a bowl, mix pomegranate seeds with yogurt and sour cream and stir.
2. Add cilantro, scallion, garlic and lemon juice and stir well again.
3. Add pepper to the taste, stir again, garnish with pomegranate seeds and serve.

Enjoy!

Nutrition: calories 182, fat 8, fiber 5, carbs 14, protein 12

Garlicky Pistachios Dip

It's such a savory party mix!

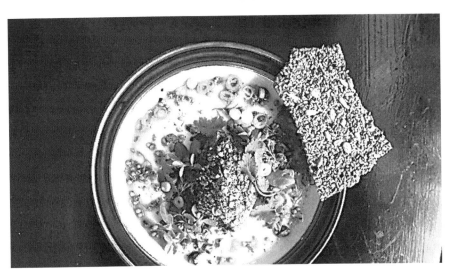

Preparation time: 10 minutes

Cooking time: 30 minutes

Servings: 6

Ingredients:

- ½ cup avocado oil
- 1 teaspoon vegetable oil
- 1 and ½ cups pistachios
- 16 garlic cloves
- ½ cup pumpkin seeds
- 1 chili pepper, chopped
- 3 scallions, chopped
- Black pepper to the taste
- 1 bunch cilantro, chopped
- 3 tablespoons lime juice
- 1 radish, sliced

Directions:

1. Heat up a pan with the oil over medium heat, add garlic, cook for 15 minutes and leave aside for now.
2. Spread pistachios and pumpkin seeds on a lined baking sheet, introduce in the oven at 350 degrees F and toast for 8 minutes.
3. Transfer ½ cup of toasted nuts and seeds to a bowl, chopped them, add pepper to the taste and a drizzle of oil and toss to coat.
4. Put the chili pepper on a lined baking sheet, introduce in the preheated broiler, broil for 10 minutes, transfer to a bowl, cover, leave aside for 15 minutes, discard seeds, peel, chop and also leave aside.
5. Heat up a pan over medium-high heat, add scallions, brown for 7 minutes stirring often, take off heat and leave aside as well.
6. In your blender, mix garlic oil with roasted chili pepper, browned scallions, lime juice the rest of the toasted nuts and seeds, cilantro, salt and pepper and pulse well.
7. Transfer dip to a bowl, sprinkle oily chopped nuts, seeds and radish and serve.

Enjoy!

Nutrition: calories 200, fat 6, fiber 5, carbs 20, protein 8

Beets Appetizer Salad

It's a colored and fresh appetizer salad!

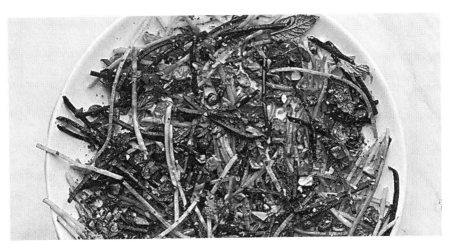

Preparation time: 10 minutes

Cooking time: 0 minutes

Servings: 4

Ingredients:

- 4 carrots, grated
- 12 radishes, grated
- 1 beet, peeled and grated
- 2 tablespoons raisins
- Juice of 2 lemons
- 1 sugar beet, peeled and chopped
- 1 tablespoon chives, chopped
- 1 tablespoon parsley, chopped
- 1 tablespoon lemon thyme, chopped
- 1 tablespoon white sesame seeds
- 4 handfuls spinach leaves
- 4 tablespoons linseed oil
- A pinch of black pepper

Directions:

1. In a salad bowl, mix carrots, radishes, beets, sugar beet, raisins, chives, parsley, spinach, thyme and sesame seeds.
2. Add lemon juice, oil and a pinch of black pepper, toss well and serve.

Enjoy!

Nutrition: calories 110, fat 4, fiber 4, carbs 8, protein 11

Artichoke Focaccia

This is so yummy!

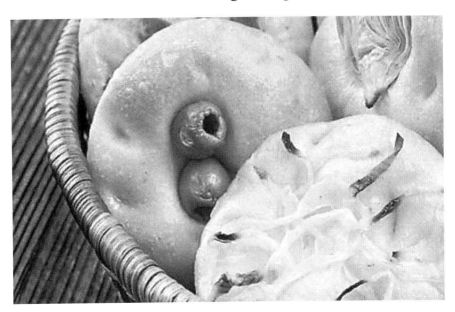

Preparation time: 10 minutes

Cooking time: 15 minutes

Servings: 1

Ingredients:

- 2 whole wheat bread shells
- 2 teaspoons olive oil
- ¼ cup artichoke hearts, chopped
- 1 tablespoon basil, chopped
- 2 tablespoons green olives, pitted and chopped
- ½ cup low-fat mozzarella cheese

Directions:

1. Rub whole wheat bread shells with the oil, sprinkle basil all over and arrange all shells on a lined baking sheet.
2. Top each focaccia with artichoke and olives, sprinkle cheese all over, introduce in the oven at 400 degrees F and bake them for 15 minutes.
3. Serve them as a snack.

Enjoy!

Nutrition: calories 152, fat 8, fiber 1, carbs 18, protein 14

Lime Crackers

These crackers are the perfect Dash diet snack!

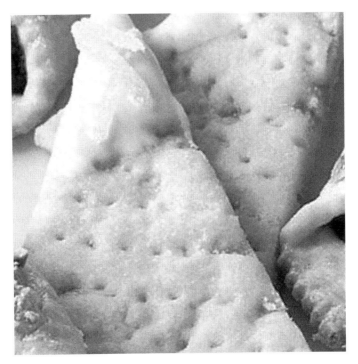

Preparation time: 10 minutes

Cooking time: 20 minutes

Servings: 4

Ingredients:

- 1 cup almond flour
- Black pepper to the taste
- 1 and ½ teaspoons lime zest
- 1 teaspoon lime juice
- 1 egg

Directions:

1. In a bowl, mix almond flour with lime zest, lime juice and stir.
2. Add egg, whisk well, divide this into 4 parts, roll each into a ball and then spread using a rolling pin.
3. Cut each into 6 triangles, place them all on a lined baking sheet, introduce in the oven at 350 degrees F and bake for 20 minutes.

Enjoy!

Nutrition: calories 90, fat 2, fiber 2, carbs 12, protein 3

Conclusion

The Dash Diet is easy as long as you follow its rules! It's a healthy lifestyle that will transform you into a healthy person in no time! The recipes I gathered for you respect the Dash Diet principles and are meant to help you with your transformation!

So, get your hands on the amazing Dash Diet cookbook, go and purchase all the ingredients you need, and get started on your new and improved life!

I am sure you will recommend this amazing diet to others as soon as you discover all its benefits!

I hope you enjoy the best life experience and have a magnificent culinary journey!

Have fun!

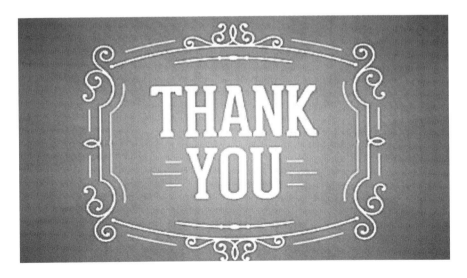

Made in the USA
Middletown, DE
02 April 2018